Disclaimer

The information contained in this book is intended for educational and informational purposes only. It is not intended as, nor should it be considered a substitute for, professional medical advice, diagnosis, or treatment. The information provided in this book should not be used for diagnosing or treating a health problem or disease. It is important to always seek the advice of a qualified healthcare provider with any questions you may have regarding a medical condition.

Self-diagnosis and self-treatment are not recommended and can be dangerous. If you have or suspect you have a medical problem, promptly contact your healthcare provider. Do not ignore professional medical advice or delay seeking medical treatment based on the information provided in this book.

The author and publisher of this book make no representation or warranties with respect to the accuracy, applicability, fitness, or completeness of the contents of this book. The author and publisher shall in no event be held liable for any loss or other damages, including but not limited to special, incidental, consequential, or other damages.

Authors Bio

Karis McRae is a purpose driven, holistic health. Fitness and mindset coach with a passion for empowering, educating and supporting others overcome negative self-perception and self-sabotaging behaviours to become their strongest, happiest, healthiest, and most confident selves!

If you would like to learn more from Karis or check out her other products, resources, and services, please visit: Linktree.com/karismcrae or email coachingwithkaris@gmail.com

Contents

Introduction	4
What is anxiety?	10
Tools for managing anxiety	13
Understanding the different types of anxiety	26
How you can support others experiencing anxiety	32
Common signs of anxiety & panic attacks	38
Reducing your anxiety	42
Recognising and managing triggers	47
The relationship between anxiety and depression	58
Social media and mental health	61
Anxiety disorders in children	65
Conclusion	69

Introduction

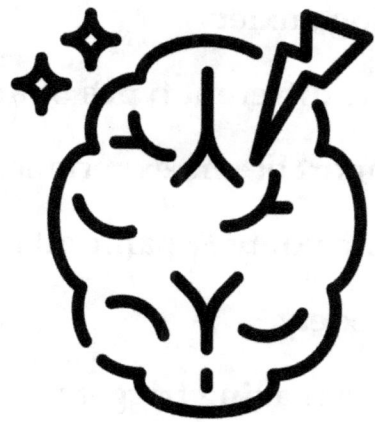

Do you ever feel a sudden tingling or numbness in your hands and feet, pressure in your chest, or fear that you may be dying or going crazy?

These are common symptoms of an anxiety attack, a condition that affects billions of people across the world.

Whether you're experiencing these symptoms yourself or know someone who is, it's important to understand anxiety and seek support.

The good news is that with understanding and support, anxiety can be managed and no longer control your life.

As a long-time sufferer of anxiety and/or depression myself as well as working with 100s of clients who too struggle with this deliberating disorder, I want to share my hope and encouragement with you.

By reading this guide, you can be empowered to help yourself and /or a loved one in their battle against anxiety. You'll learn that you're not alone in your struggles, as there are countless others who are struggling also.

So, if you're feeling overwhelmed by anxiety, know that you can get help and overcome this affliction. You can learn to live with it and stop giving it the power to control you.

The first step is to seek support and to educate yourself so that you fully understand what anxiety is.

My goal is to give you the tools and support you need to feel empowered and confident in your journey to managing anxiety.

Remember, you are not alone!

Anxiety Disorders – An Overwhelming Experience

Anxiety disorders can be a challenging and overwhelming experience, especially during periods of high stress.

It's not uncommon for those with anxiety disorders to also struggle with symptoms of depression. To address this, treatment options often involve a combination of therapy, lifestyle changes, and medication. However, it's important to note that what works best for one person may not work for another, as everyone's circumstances, genetics, and lifestyles are unique.

Mainstream treatment typically involves prescription medication and therapy, but the efficacy of this combination is a topic of debate in the medical community. Some studies show that the combination is more effective than either approach alone, while others indicate that medication may provide greater relief than therapy.

To determine the best course of action, it's essential to work with a trusted mental health professional, such as a counsellor, therapist, or coach, who can take into account your individual circumstances and lifestyle.

In some cases, making simple lifestyle changes, such as adopting a nutrient-rich, low-processed food diet and incorporating exercise, may be all that's needed to experience significant improvement. So, if you or someone you know is struggling with anxiety disorders, don't give up hope. There is support available, and together with the right professional guidance, it's possible to find a treatment plan that works for you.

Who Is Affected By Anxiety?

Anxiety is a prevalent disorder that can affect anyone, regardless of age, social status, or background. It's not uncommon to see friends, family members, or even public figures suffering from anxiety in silence, as the stigma surrounding mental health often leads to feelings of shame and embarrassment.

As a result, many people hide their struggles, which can exacerbate their symptoms and make them feel isolated.

Despite this, it's essential to remember that anxiety is not a reflection of someone's strength or character. It's a real health condition that can be caused by a combination of genetic and environmental factors.

Many famous artists, actors, and comedians have also faced challenges with anxiety and depression, often successfully keeping it hidden from the public view and even their loved ones.

If you or someone you know is struggling with anxiety, it's crucial to reach out for help.

A combination of medication, therapy, and lifestyle changes can help manage the symptoms and improve overall well-being. Working with a mental health professional can help identify the best treatment plan and provide support during the healing process.

Here's some interesting statistical facts for you:

1. There were 8.2 million cases of anxiety in the UK in 2013 (1) 2 Women are twice as likely to be diagnosed with anxiety (2,3) 3 7.2% of 5–19-year-olds experience an anxiety condition (4) 4 In 2017, 3.9% of 5–10-year-old children had an anxiety disorder, as did 7.5% of 11–16-year-olds and 13.1% of 17–19-year-olds (4).

2. Among those aged 17-19, 10.1% had a probably mental disorder in 2017, rising to 17.4% in 2021. Rates remained similar between 2020 and 2021.

3. Among those aged 17-19, 10.1% had a probably mental disorder in 2017, rising to 17.4% in 2021. Rates remained similar between 2020 and 2021.

4. In the UK, over 8 million people are experiencing an anxiety disorder at any one time (Mental Health UK) Less than 50% of people with generalised anxiety disorder access treatment (Mental Health Foundation) An estimated 822,000 workers are affected by work-related stress, depression or anxiety every year (Health and Safety Executive)

Coincidentally, the major reason for people not knowing what is happening to them, or that they are suffering from Anxiety or panic disorder could be attributed to the fact that many cases reported began in adolescence.

Therefore, a child may not be as affluent in describing what they are experiencing compared to the ability of that of an adult.

The key here is to listen to your children!

You would not want them to endure a childhood full of suffering and not even know the reason for it. Another interesting fact to be aware of is that Anxiety attacks don't only happen when a person is awake! They can, and often do, happen while sleeping. How scary do you think that may be to wake up to? Indescribable would be putting it mildly.

What Is Anxiety?

Imagine being in a situation where you are standing in front of a speeding train, frozen to the spot and unable to move, knowing that there's absolutely nothing you can do to escape.

Now imagine going through this scenario multiple times a day. This is what it feels like for someone with anxiety disorder. The fear they experience is intense, irrational, and overwhelming, often leaving them with a sense of dread and doom.

Unlike a speeding train, this fear is unseen and comes from nowhere, striking at any moment of the day.

Anxiety disorder is characterized by feelings of intense, irrational fear. This means that for someone suffering from anxiety disorder, they may be hit with paralysing fear for no apparent reason, making them feel like there is no escape. Unfortunately, anxiety disorder often co-occurs with other mental health conditions such as depression, obsessive-compulsive disorder, agoraphobia, and phobias, which highlights the importance of seeking treatment.

Understanding The Causes of Anxiety

The truth is, Anxiety can be influenced by a variety of things, and sometimes seemingly nothing at all! Many times, Anxiety is brought about due to increased stress from daily life. Bills piling up, children spiraling out of control, pressure from work, family, and other events can trigger this disorder bringing it to the surface of an otherwise "dormant" carrier of the genetic traits passed on by their parents.

At its core, anxiety is a product of the mind, with the brain playing a central role in its manifestation. Scientific studies have pinpointed two specific areas of the brain that are responsible for generating feelings of fear and anxiety. When triggered, these areas activate the body's "fight or flight" defense mechanism, releasing adrenaline and sending the sufferer into a full-blown anxiety attack.

Many people develop anxiety as a result of increased stress in their daily lives. This can include anything from financial pressure to family problems, and it can bring an otherwise "dormant" anxiety disorder to the surface. For these people, the fear of an anxiety attack can be a vicious cycle, with the memory of past attacks triggering new ones.

While it is true that anxiety is "all in your mind," this statement can come across as dismissive or condescending to those who suffer from the condition. The truth is, anxiety is a real and debilitating condition that requires proper treatment and support.

Tools For Managing Anxiety

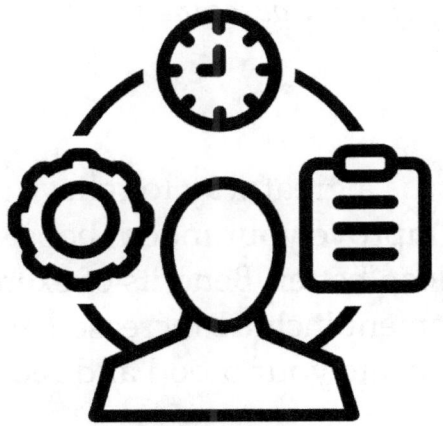

Anxiety can be a normal and expected aspect of life, but for those who experience an anxiety disorder, it can quickly spiral out of control and become overwhelming. However, there is hope for those struggling with anxiety as there are numerous ways to tackle it and reduce its impact on daily life. By taking small, yet meaningful steps, you can learn how to manage your anxiety and regain control over your thoughts and emotions.

This can involve seeking professional help, developing healthy coping mechanisms, practicing self-care, and making changes to your lifestyle to reduce stress and promote overall well-being. Remember, taking control of your anxiety is possible, and you don't have to face it alone.

Here are some simple, yet highly effective things you can begin implementing into your daily life to help you manage and hopefully overcome your anxiety:

Exercise:

Regular exercise is a great way to relieve stress and anxiety. It can improve your mood, boost self-esteem, and help you sleep better. Benefits of exercise for anxiety management include increased endorphins, which help to elevate your mood and reduce feelings of anxiety.
Negatives of not engaging in regular exercise include increased stress levels and a decreased ability to manage anxiety.

Caffeine:

Consuming caffeine can increase feelings of anxiety and nervousness. To help manage anxiety, it is recommended to limit or avoid caffeine. Benefits of reducing caffeine intake include reduced nervousness, improved sleep, and a calmer state of mind.
Negatives of not reducing caffeine intake include increased anxiety, poor sleep, and disrupted hormone levels.

Positive Affirmations:

Positive affirmations can help you shift your focus from negative thoughts and beliefs to positive ones.

Benefits of positive affirmations include increased self-confidence, reduced anxiety, and improved overall mood. Negatives of not using positive affirmations include a lack of focus on positive thoughts, increased anxiety, and decreased self-confidence.

Examples:

"I am in control of my thoughts and emotions."
"I am strong and capable of handling any situation that comes my way."
"I trust in my abilities to overcome anxiety."
"I am worthy of peace and happiness."
"I am deserving of a calm and balanced life."

<u>Sleep:</u>

Getting enough sleep is crucial for managing anxiety. Poor sleep can lead to increased feelings of anxiety and decreased ability to manage it. Benefits of getting enough sleep include reduced stress, improved mood, and better overall mental health.
Negatives of not getting enough sleep include increased anxiety, poor mental health, and decreased ability to manage stress.

<u>Controlled Breathing:</u>

Controlled breathing is a great way to calm down during moments of anxiety.

It can help slow your heart rate, reduce feelings of stress, and improve your overall sense of well-being. Benefits of controlled breathing include reduced anxiety, improved mental clarity, and increased relaxation. Negatives of not practicing controlled breathing include increased anxiety and stress, decreased ability to manage anxiety, and poor mental clarity.

Stress Management:

Managing stress is crucial for managing anxiety. High levels of stress can trigger or worsen anxiety symptoms. Benefits of managing stress include reduced anxiety, improved mental health, and better overall quality of life.
Negatives of not managing stress include increased anxiety, poor mental health, and decreased ability to live a fulfilling life.

Anxiety can leave you feeling burdened and overcome and defeated. By taking these simple measures, you can begin to manage and reduce the severity of anxiety symptoms and effectively take back control.

Relieving Your Anxiety

Anxiety is a vicious cycle that can leave an individual feeling trapped in a never-ending loop of negative thoughts and emotions. The feeling of anxiety is intense and overwhelming and can trigger a series of events that only amplifies its effects. This, in turn, leads to an increase in the level of anxiety, leaving the individual feeling helpless and powerless.

The fear and nervousness that anxiety brings on is overwhelming, and it can be difficult to break free from this cycle, especially when the feeling only seems to get worse with time. This cycle can make it challenging to think rationally and cope with the situation effectively, which can lead to feelings of desperation and hopelessness.

If you suffer from anxiety attacks regularly, here are some effective things you can try to start to relieve your anxiety:

1. Making yourself Comfortable:

It is important to be in a comfortable environment when experiencing anxiety.

This can mean different things to different people, but some tips include making sure the room temperature is comfortable, wearing comfortable clothing, and having a comfortable place to sit.

The goal is to create a physical environment that helps reduce physical tension, which can make the mind feel more relaxed.

Benefits:

Creating a comfortable physical environment can help reduce physical tension and therefore reduce feelings of anxiety. This can be especially helpful for those who experience physical symptoms such as sweating, shaking, or rapid heartbeat.

Negative Effect of Not Doing So:

If you are not in a comfortable physical environment, this can contribute to feelings of anxiety and make symptoms worse.

2. Empowering Self Talk:

The things we say to ourselves can greatly impact our emotions and thoughts. It is important to engage in positive self-talk when experiencing anxiety. This can involve speaking out loud or silently repeating affirmations that you believe about yourself.

Benefits:

Engaging in positive self-talk can help change your thoughts and reduce feelings of anxiety. This can help you feel more in control and improve your overall mood.

Negative Effect of Not Doing So:

Negative self-talk can contribute to feelings of anxiety and make symptoms worse.

3. Relaxation Techniques:

Relaxation techniques such as deep breathing, progressive muscle relaxation, and guided imagery can help to reduce feelings of anxiety. These techniques can be learned and practiced regularly to help manage anxiety symptoms.

Benefits:

Relaxation techniques can help reduce physical and emotional tension, which can help reduce feelings of anxiety. Practicing these techniques regularly can help you feel more in control and improve your overall mood.

Negative Effect of Not Doing So:

If you do not engage in relaxation techniques, this can contribute to feelings of anxiety and make symptoms worse.

4. Acknowledging Anxious Thoughts:

It is important to acknowledge your anxious thoughts and not try to ignore or suppress them.
Try to recognize that these thoughts are a normal part of the anxiety experience and do not define who you are.

Benefits:

Acknowledging anxious thoughts can help you gain a sense of control over them and reduce feelings of anxiety. This can help you feel more in control and improve your overall mood.

Negative Effect of Not Doing So:

Ignoring or suppressing anxious thoughts can contribute to feelings of anxiety and make symptoms worse.

5. Distracting Yourself with Other Things:

Finding a distraction that you enjoy can help to reduce feelings of anxiety.
This can involve engaging in activities such as reading, watching a movie, playing a game, or doing a hobby.

Benefits:

Engaging in a distraction can help take your mind off of anxious thoughts and reduce feelings of anxiety. This can help you feel more in control and improve your overall mood.

Negative Effect of Not Doing So:

If you do not engage in distractions, this can contribute to feelings of anxiety and make symptoms worse.

Natural Remedies For Managing Anxiety

Natural remedies, such as herbs, diet, and supplements, have been used for centuries to manage and treat various health conditions, including anxiety.

These alternative treatments offer a more holistic approach to managing anxiety symptoms and can be a great option for those who are looking to avoid prescription medication or for those who are seeking a more natural way to manage their condition.
Herbs such as chamomile, passionflower, and kava are often used for their calming effects and to help relieve anxiety symptoms.

Additionally, certain supplements such as magnesium, probiotics, and omega-3 fatty acids have been shown to have a positive impact on mental health and can help reduce symptoms of anxiety. A healthy and balanced diet can also play a key role in managing anxiety, as what you eat can affect your mood and energy levels.

By making simple changes to your lifestyle and incorporating these natural remedies, you can help reduce your symptoms of anxiety and achieve a better state of mental well-being.

Herbs

Chamomile:
Chamomile tea has been used for centuries as a natural remedy for anxiety.
Chamomile contains compounds that can act as a mild sedative, helping to calm the mind and reduce anxiety symptoms.

Valerian Root:
Valerian root is another herb that is often used as a natural remedy for anxiety.
It is thought to act as a natural tranquilizer, helping to reduce feelings of anxiety and improve sleep quality.

Passionflower:
Passionflower is an herb that has been used for centuries to treat anxiety, nervousness, and insomnia. It contains compounds that can help to calm the mind and reduce anxiety symptoms.

Lavender:

Lavender is an herb that is often used as an aromatherapy treatment for anxiety.
The scent of lavender has been shown to help reduce stress and anxiety levels, while also improving mood and promoting relaxation.

Benefits: Using herbs as a natural treatment for anxiety can be a safe and effective alternative to medication. They are typically non-addictive, have few side effects, and can be taken alongside other medications if needed.

Supplements

Omega-3 Fatty Acids:
Omega-3 fatty acids are essential fatty acids that have been shown to have a positive impact on mental health, including reducing anxiety symptoms.

Magnesium:
Magnesium is a mineral that is essential for good health. Research has found that magnesium deficiencies are linked to increased levels of anxiety and depression, making it an important supplement for anxiety sufferers.

B-complex vitamins:
B-complex vitamins, particularly vitamin B6 and vitamin B12, have been shown to have a positive impact on mood and mental health, including reducing anxiety symptoms.

Ashwagandha:
Ashwagandha is an adaptogenic herb that is used in Ayurvedic medicine to help reduce stress and anxiety levels.
It works by modulating cortisol levels in the body, which can help to reduce feelings of stress and anxiety.

Benefits:
Supplements can provide an additional source of nutrients that can help support your overall mental health, reducing anxiety symptoms. They can also be a convenient and easy way to get the nutrients your body needs without having to make major changes to your diet.

Diet

Eating a balanced and healthy diet that includes plenty of fresh fruits and vegetables, lean proteins, and healthy fats can help to support good mental health and reduce anxiety symptoms.

Avoiding caffeine, alcohol, and processed foods can also be helpful, as these substances can trigger or worsen anxiety symptoms.

Benefits: Making changes to your diet to support good mental health can help to reduce anxiety symptoms and improve your overall health and well-being.
By focusing on eating a balanced and nutritious diet, you can help to keep your body and mind healthy, reducing the impact of anxiety on your life.

Blood Sugar

Maintaining stable blood sugar levels can be helpful for managing anxiety symptoms. Eating a diet that is high in refined carbohydrates, sugar, and processed foods can cause spikes and crashes in blood sugar levels, which can trigger anxiety symptoms.

Eating regular, balanced meals and snacks that include a mix of complex carbohydrates, proteins, and healthy fats can help to regulate blood sugar levels and reduce anxiety symptoms.

Benefits: Regulating blood sugar levels can be a key component of treating anxiety naturally. By maintaining stable blood sugar levels, you can help to reduce feelings of stress and anxiety, while also improving your overall health and well-being.

Discovering natural ways to manage anxiety without relying on prescription drugs can have a significant impact in reducing your anxiety symptoms. With a few modifications to your daily habits, you can overcome anxiety and reclaim control of your life.

Understanding the different Types of Anxiety

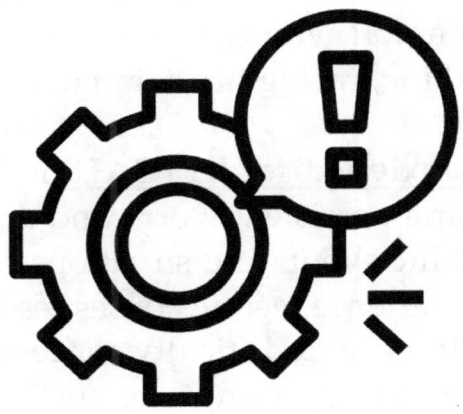

Did you know that there are several distinct varieties of anxiety? In this initial section, we will delve into the different types of anxiety.

Anxiety is a complex and multi-faceted experience that can take on many different forms. Understanding the different types of anxiety can help people better identify their specific symptoms and find the best way to manage their anxiety.

Social anxiety disorder is characterised by intense fear and self-consciousness in social situations.

People with social anxiety disorder often feel highly anxious and self-conscious around others, fearing that they will be judged, criticised, or embarrassed. They may avoid social situations or engage in them with great difficulty. Common symptoms include blushing, sweating, shaking, racing heart and dry mouth.

<u>Generalised anxiety disorder (GAD)</u> is characterized by excessive and persistent worry and anxiety about a wide range of life events and situations. People with GAD often experience feelings of restlessness, irritability, fatigue, and difficulty concentrating. They may also have physical symptoms such as headaches, muscle tension, and digestive problems. GAD can interfere with daily life and make it difficult to go about normal activities.

<u>Panic disorder and panic attacks</u> are characterized by sudden, intense, and unexpected episodes of fear, along with physical symptoms such as racing heart, sweating, shaking, chest pain, and shortness of breath. Panic attacks often occur without any clear trigger and can be very distressing and frightening. People with panic disorder may avoid situations where they have had panic attacks or live in constant fear of having another one.

In all of these types of anxiety, the feelings, symptoms, and effects can be highly individualised.

They can range from mild to severe and may last for varying amounts of time. However, one common thread is that anxiety can have a profound impact on a person's quality of life, making it difficult for them to engage in normal activities, form relationships, and maintain a sense of well-being.

The key to managing and reducing anxiety is to understand the different types and find the most effective strategies for treating each individual case. This may involve a combination of lifestyle changes, therapy, medications, and other treatments, as well as the use of self-help techniques and support from family and friends.

Things You Can Do To Help Overcome Anxiety Attacks

It is important to recognize an anxiety attack for what it is when you are experiencing one. Realize that it is only a temporary episode and that it will eventually pass. Anxiety attacks typically last from a few minutes to a maximum of 30 minutes.

To ease the symptoms, try to find a comfortable position, whether it be lying down or sitting still, and focus on slow, even breathing. This can help you get through the attack.

The key to overcoming anxiety is to redirect your thoughts and keep yourself occupied. By doing so, the fear and thoughts of an impending attack will gradually fade away. With practice, you will become more proficient at managing anxiety attacks.

If you find that you are unable to manage the attack on your own, don't hesitate to seek medical help. Emergency services are trained to handle these situations and there is no need to feel ashamed or embarrassed.

How To Prepare For Potential Anxiety attacks

Anxiety is a common mental health condition that affects millions of people worldwide. Anxiety attacks can be sudden and intense, causing physical and emotional distress.

Preparation is key in managing anxiety attacks and can greatly reduce their frequency and intensity. Here are five ways people with anxiety can prepare in advance:

1. Identifying triggers:

Understanding what triggers your anxiety attacks is a crucial step in preparation.

Common triggers include stressful events, certain environments, or even specific thoughts. Identifying these triggers can help you avoid or prepare for them.

2. Coping strategies:

Having a set of coping strategies can be incredibly helpful during an anxiety attack.
These can include deep breathing exercises, mindfulness, or physical activity. Practicing these strategies in advance can make them more automatic and effective when an attack occurs.

3. Developing a support network:

Having a supportive network of friends, family, or mental health professionals can be invaluable in managing anxiety attacks. Sharing your experiences with loved ones can help them understand your needs and provide comfort during an attack.

4. Mindful self-care:

Taking care of your physical and emotional health can help prevent anxiety attacks from occurring or reduce their severity.
This can include regular exercise, a balanced diet, and getting enough sleep.

Relaxation techniques:

Relaxation techniques, such as progressive muscle relaxation or guided imagery, can help reduce anxiety and stress. Practicing these techniques regularly can help you stay calm during an anxiety attack.

Preparing in advance for anxiety attacks can help you feel more in control and reduce the frequency and intensity of these events. It can also increase your overall well-being and reduce the impact of anxiety on your daily life. By taking proactive steps, you can increase your resilience and manage your anxiety more effectively.

How You Can Support Others Experiencing Anxiety

As we go through this information, I want you to understand that this section is of importance to those trying to help another person who is experiencing, or dealing with, Anxiety on a daily basis.

How you provide support to them may help them to control their Anxiety to some degree.

First thing is first. Never belittle or try to downplay someone's anxiety disorder. This is a real disorder and should be respected as such. Don't just dismiss their episode as a onetime event or try and 'solve' their problem through rationalisation.

You must understand that when a person is actually going through an Anxiety attack rationality is not something they are concentrating on or listening to.

This is an extremely frightening experience and no matter how much you'd want to, you cannot make this experience go away. Only the individual who is having the attack has the power to do this, not you.

The absolute worst thing you can do is to act as if they are lying or acting to get attention. This is simply not the case. While you may BELIEVE this to be true because you have never yourself experienced the unrelenting terror of an Anxiety attack, that doesn't mean that it isn't happening to someone you care about.

Imagine for a second that you had witnessed a "physical" accident that your loved one or dear friend was a part of. Something you could see the outcome from. Wouldn't you do everything in your power to help them?

What if they were trapped inside a car that was on fire? What if they were trapped underwater and were drowning? You would want to aid them, wouldn't you? What if they had stopped breathing? Would you just stand around watching them pass away? Or would you do everything you could to administer CPR to them, even if you weren't sure, you were doing it correctly?

While the above examples are extreme, sometimes, to an anxiety sufferer, it absolutely feels like the end of their world. As if they are drowning in a sea of chaos and disparity, unable to pull themselves out.

Also, by attempting to in effect ignore the Anxiety attack, you are probably contributing to another disorder that goes hand in hand with anxiety and depression.

Instead of holding them down 'under water,' try throwing them a life preserver the next time they have an attack.

How can you do that? Just be there for them. Let them know that while you may not understand what they are going through, you are there for them and will stay until they feel better.

Don't ever try and force someone out of an Anxiety attack. It could make the attack that much worse for them. Just let the attack happen naturally, and in most, if not all, cases, their bodies will help them come out of the 'hot' zone all on its own. If it doesn't, get them to the nearest A&E as soon as you can.

Also, never try and give someone suffering from an anxiety attack any type of prescription medication that have not been prescribed by their Doctor or a medical professional.

This may seem like common sense, but when you see a loved one experiencing such a destressing event, you really want to help them. Believe me, this will not help them. Getting them to a professional source, such as an emergency room or their own family physician, for help WILL.

Seeking Professional Support For Anxiety

If you have exhausted all your own mental power to overcome Anxiety on your own, there is still help for you. The best course of action for you at this point is to seek out professional help through your trusted health professional.

They will inform you on what you should do and the best steps for you to take to have fulfilling life without it being completely taken over and controlled by your Anxiety.

If you don't have a family Doctor, you can still get help for Anxiety through your local area mental health facilities. There are a lot of places that are equipped to deal with many different mental health disorders and illnesses, one of which is anxiety and panic disorder and can be identified relatively easily through a simple Google search.

Never think that you are going through this alone. There are millions of other people struggling with Anxiety just as you are every single day.

There are support groups, counselling services you should take advantage of, anxiety related programs to help you make sense of and learn to control your Anxiety, and of course there are effective medicines your doctor can prescribe for you if necessary.

Anxiety Disorders: What Are They & How To Diagnose Them In Yourself & Loved Ones

Anxiety disorders are a group of mental health conditions characterized by excessive and persistent feelings of fear, worry, and unease. These feelings can be so severe that they interfere with daily activities, including work, school, and relationships. The most common types of anxiety disorders are:

1. Generalized Anxiety Disorder (GAD): This type of anxiety disorder is characterized by excessive and persistent worry about everyday events and activities. People with GAD may have physical symptoms such as headaches, muscle tension, and fatigue.

2. Panic Disorder:
This type of anxiety disorder is characterized by sudden and intense feelings of fear, called panic attacks. Panic attacks can be triggered by specific objects or situations, or they can happen without any apparent trigger.

3. Social Anxiety Disorder (SAD):
This type of anxiety disorder is characterized by intense fear and self-consciousness in social situations. People with SAD may worry about being embarrassed, judged, or rejected.

4. Phobias:
Phobias are intense and irrational fears of specific objects or situations, such as heights, spiders, or flying. People with phobias avoid the objects or situations they fear, which can limit their daily activities.

5. Post-Traumatic Stress Disorder (PTSD):
This type of anxiety disorder can develop after a person experiences or witnesses a traumatic event, such as a natural disaster, war, or sexual assault. People with PTSD may experience flashbacks, nightmares, and feelings of guilt, shame, or fear.

To diagnose an anxiety disorder, a mental health professional will conduct a thorough evaluation, including a medical history, a psychological evaluation, and a review of symptoms. They may also use standardized questionnaires and assessments to help determine the presence of an anxiety disorder.

If you suspect that you or a loved one may have an anxiety disorder, it's important to seek help from a mental health professional. Treatment for anxiety disorders can include therapy, medication, and lifestyle changes. With the right support and treatment, it's possible to manage symptoms and improve quality of life.

Common Signs of Anxiety & Panic Attacks

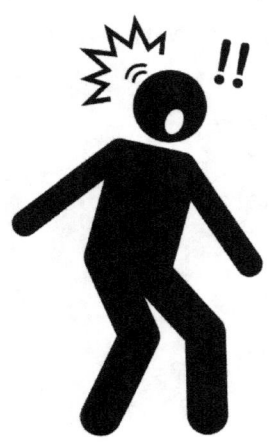

You don't need to have a diagnosis of an anxiety disorder to suffer from an anxiety attack, they don't discriminate and can strike anyone.

Panic attacks are sudden and intense feelings of fear and anxiety that can be overwhelming. They can occur with or without a clear trigger and can last anywhere from a few minutes to several hours.

The signs and symptoms of a panic attack can be broadly classified into three categories: emotional, psychological, and physical.

Emotional symptoms of a panic attack include:

1. Fear:
People with panic attacks often experience intense and irrational fear, which can feel like a sense of impending doom.

2. Anxiety:
People with panic attacks often feel anxious and worried, even when there is no immediate threat.

3. Nervousness:
People with panic attacks often feel nervous and jittery, as if something bad is about to happen.

Psychological symptoms of a panic attack include:

1. Uncontrollable thoughts:
People with panic attacks may have thoughts that are intrusive and difficult to control, such as fear of losing control or going crazy.

2. Mental confusion:

People with panic attacks may feel mentally confused and disoriented, making it difficult to focus or make decisions.

3. Perception of reality:
People with panic attacks may perceive reality differently during a panic attack, and feel as if they are detached from the world around them.

Physical symptoms of a panic attack include:

1. Rapid heartbeat:
People with panic attacks may experience a rapid heartbeat, which can feel like their heart is racing or pounding.

5. Shortness of breath:
People with panic attacks may feel short of breath or as if they are suffocating.

6. Chest pain:
People with panic attacks may experience chest pain or tightness, which can feel like a heart attack.

7. Sweating:
People with panic attacks may sweat profusely, even in cool environments.

8. Shaking or trembling:
People with panic attacks may shake or tremble, which can feel like a physical expression of their inner fear.

9. Nausea:
People with panic attacks may feel nauseous or experience digestive distress, such as abdominal pain or diarrhea.

10. Dizziness:
People with panic attacks may feel dizzy or lightheaded, as if they are about to faint.

It's important to note that not everyone with panic attacks will experience all of these symptoms, and that the symptoms can vary from person to person and from attack to attack. If you experience panic attacks and are concerned about your symptoms, it's important to seek help from a mental health professional.

Reducing Your Anxiety

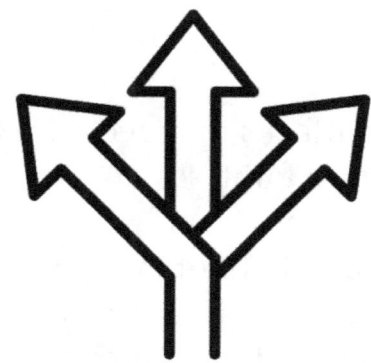

If your fears and anxiety are holding you back from living the life you want, you're not alone.

In the UK, over **8 million people** are experiencing an anxiety disorder at any one time. The good news is that there are studies that show by facing your fears you can gain the courage you need to overcome other concerns that you may have.

Here are some tips for facing your fears and overcoming anxiety:

Don't Go It Alone:
When you are facing down your fears, it can be beneficial to have someone along for the journey that can cheer you on.

Perhaps you know someone who has the same fear as you, that can partner with you so that you can encourage and cheer each other on.

Boost Your Confidence:
When you are getting ready to stare down your fear, it can be immensely helpful to remember all the other courageous things that you've accomplished in your life. Remember how it felt to achieve your goal. Recognizing previous acts of courage can go a long way in helping you face your fears.

Acknowledge The Fear:
Many times, our fears are relegated to the back of our minds, unacknowledged and ignored. Even when faced with anxiety, we often choose just to feel the issue, and never really take the time to understand our fear.

Start paying attention to how your body feels and acknowledge the sensation as a symptom rather than something more significant.

Keep a Gratitude Journal:
There have been many studies over the years on the positive effects of keeping a gratitude journal.

These studies suggest that people who practice gratitude had higher levels of positive emotions, a stronger immune system, felt less lonely, and had more happiness in their lives. Rather than focusing on the negative in your life, be thankful for everything that you have.

Expose Yourself To What You Fear:
Even though it can be terrifying, if you want to overcome your fears, then you must face them. Sit down and define the worst-case scenario of the unknown outcome, an realize that the worst scenario rarely happens.

Doing this you'll start to notice that each time you do the scary thing, it gets a little bit easier.

It is possible to face your fears and overcome your anxiety. Facing your fear will lead you to live a better life, free from stress and anxiety.

Important Steps To Stop Your Anxiety

When excessive fears and worries plague you, it is critical to figure out what you can do to stop the anxiety so that it doesn't completely take over your life.

If you have an anxiety disorder, it's essential that you find simple strategies that can help you manage or reduce your anxiety.

Here are some things that you can do now to help stop your anxiety before it gets out of control:

Understand The Anatomy Of Your Anxiety:
When you understand what your anxiety attack is, what causes them, and how your body responds, you can keep from becoming scared of the symptoms.

When you can become unafraid of your anxiety symptoms, you can quickly put a stop to them when your mind starts to race with anxious thoughts. Knowledge is power, and the more you can understand your anxiety, the faster you can stop it from controlling your life.

Stop Scaring Yourself:
Fear is the most common culprits behind anxiety. When you can refuse to allow, yourself to become scared you can effectively remove the primary reason for your anxiety.
When you eliminate fear from your life, you can gain more control of your body's emergency response system and take control of your anxiety.

Calm Yourself:
Being able to calm yourself down helps to shut off the mechanism in your brain that causes anxiety attacks and ends your body's stress response.

The more you can calm yourself down, the faster you can stop the anxiety attack and start to feel better. A sure way to end, control, and prevent future panic attacks is to find out ways to calm yourself down.

Distract Yourself:
Most anxiety attacks are caused and fueled by anxious thoughts. When you can distract your attention, you can effectively prevent anxious thoughts from taking over. As you prevent your thoughts from turning anxious, you can also put an end to voluntary anxiety attacks.

Know That Anxiety Attacks End:
No matter how powerful an anxiety attack can be, it will always end. While you can stop them faster by implementing some of the above techniques and methods, you must remember that all anxiety attacks will end.

Riding out the anxiety attack and knowing that it will end, can help you to stay calm and shut off the stress response and anxiety attack. You don't need to suffer needlessly. You can eliminate your anxiety attacks naturally with these simple tips.

Recognising and Managing Triggers

Anxiety disorders are incredibly common, as are many of the things that will trigger anxiety.

For most people dealing with anxiety, they find that they have multiple triggers, while other people's anxiety attacks are triggered for no reason at all.

If you want to gain control of your anxiety, it's important to discover any triggers that you may have. Triggers are events, situations, or experiences that can cause a sudden increase in anxiety or other emotional distress. Triggers can be physical, emotional, or a combination of both, and they can vary from person to person.
Understanding your triggers and learning to manage them is an important step in managing anxiety and other mental health conditions.

Physical Triggers:

Physical triggers are events or stimuli that affect the body, such as changes in temperature, hunger, or fatigue. Examples of physical triggers include:

1. Illness: Being sick or experiencing pain can trigger feelings of anxiety and stress, especially if the illness or pain is chronic.

2. Sleep deprivation: Lack of sleep can increase feelings of stress and anxiety, making it important to get enough rest each night.

3. Diet: Consuming foods high in sugar, caffeine, or artificial preservatives can trigger anxiety and other physical symptoms.

Emotional Triggers:

Emotional triggers are events or stimuli that affect the emotions, such as memories, thoughts, or relationships. Examples of emotional triggers include:

1. Stressful events: Major life events, such as moving, losing a job, or ending a relationship, can trigger feelings of anxiety and stress.

2. Negative thoughts: Thoughts and beliefs that are negative, such as self-doubt, can trigger feelings of anxiety and stress.

3. Trauma: Traumatic experiences, such as abuse, neglect, or natural disasters, can trigger feelings of anxiety and post-traumatic stress disorder (PTSD).

Managing Triggers:

There are several strategies for managing triggers, both mental and physical, including:

1. Mindfulness: Practicing mindfulness can help you become more aware of your thoughts, emotions, and physical sensations, which can make it easier to manage triggers.

2. Relaxation techniques: Relaxation techniques, such as deep breathing, progressive muscle relaxation, and yoga, can help you manage physical symptoms of anxiety and stress.

3. Cognitive-behavioural therapy (CBT): CBT is a type of therapy that can help you change negative thoughts and beliefs, making it easier to manage emotional triggers.
4. Exercise: Exercise can help you manage physical symptoms of anxiety and stress, as well as release endorphins that can improve mood.

5. Healthy habits: Maintaining a healthy diet, getting enough sleep, and avoiding substances that can trigger anxiety, such as caffeine, can help you manage triggers and maintain good mental health.

Conclusion

Triggers are a common part of life, but they can be difficult to manage when they trigger feelings of anxiety and stress. Understanding your triggers and learning to manage them can help you maintain good mental health and prevent anxiety from affecting your daily life. Whether you choose to manage your triggers through mindfulness, therapy, exercise, or healthy habits, the key is to find what works for you and stick with it.

Learn To Manage Your Anxiety

It's estimated over **8 million people** are experiencing an anxiety disorder at any one time in the UK alone, which makes it the most common mental illness in the country. Anxiety can impact anyone, regardless of the kind of life they lead.

Unfortunately, many people suffer in silence because they are ashamed to admit their struggles with anxiety.

If you are one of the millions who suffer from anxiety, here are some useful tips to help you better manage your condition:

Watch For Your Triggers:

If you know what triggers your anxiety, you can then effectively plan your day around them.
If there are times throughout the day that you know your anxiety is likely to be triggered, plan time-outs, or periods of exercise during these times. Understanding your danger spots can help to lessen your anxiety.

Start Exercising:

Regular daily exercise has many benefits, including helping to alleviate the debilitating symptoms of anxiety. If you haven't made regular exercise a habit in your life, its time you start.

You don't have to spend hours in the gym, even a short walk around the block every day can significantly impact your life and decrease your anxiety.

Take Some Time To Breathe:

When your symptoms of anxiety start to rear their ugly head, taking some time alone to breathe can be highly effective in managing your anxiety. Deep breathing exercises can help to calm your heart and help you instantly feel at peace. It can also aid in our ability to make rational decisions.

Talk To Someone You Trust:
You don't have to suffer in silence. Reach out to someone who will treat you with understanding and kindness.
If you don't have any support at home, or with friends, then you can look up local support groups near your home or place of business. There are always resources available, all you have to do is reach out.

Understand That You're in Control:
While it may not feel this way when you're in the midst of a panic attack, it is essential to understand that you have the power of your life.
Even if you feel trapped, or out of control, you have to realise that you have control over every decision that you make in your life.

You don't have to let your anxiety rule your life. Incorporate these tips into your life daily and take control of your anxiety and take back your life.

Foods That Can Influence Anxiety

You are probably already aware that your emotions can significantly influence what you eat. However, as outlined briefly previously, did you also know that what you eat can dramatically affect your mood?

If you didn't already know, some foods could worsen your anxiety. According to research conducted by Harvard Health, simple food choices can make a significant difference in how you feel.

Diet plays a crucial role in our overall health and wellbeing, and this includes our mental health. The food we consume can have a direct impact on the way we feel and think. Our diets can either improve or worsen our mental health and mood.
Today, our diets are heavily influenced by convenience and fast-paced lifestyles, leading to an overproduction of processed foods and an increased reliance on unhealthy food options. These types of foods often contain high amounts of sugar, unhealthy fats, and artificial ingredients, all of which can have a negative impact on our mental health.

Studies have shown that consuming high amounts of sugar and unhealthy fats can contribute to the development of depression, anxiety, and other mental health conditions. These types of foods have been linked to the imbalance of neurotransmitters in the brain, leading to an increased risk of developing mental health disorders.

On the other hand, a diet rich in fruits, vegetables, whole grains, and lean proteins has been shown to have a positive impact on mental health. These types of foods contain essential vitamins and minerals, such as omega-3 fatty acids, which are important for brain function and mental health. They also provide the body with the energy it needs to function properly, reducing the risk of mental health conditions.

Studies have shown that consuming high amounts of sugar and unhealthy fats can contribute to the development of depression, anxiety, and other mental health conditions. These types of foods have been linked to the imbalance of neurotransmitters in the brain, leading to an increased risk of developing mental health disorders.

On the other hand, a diet rich in fruits, vegetables, whole grains, and lean proteins has been shown to have a positive impact on mental health.

These types of foods contain essential vitamins and minerals, such as omega-3 fatty acids, which are important for brain function and mental health. They also provide the body with the energy it needs to function properly, reducing the risk of mental health conditions.

Here are some specific foods that you should avoid if you suffer from Anxiety:

Processed Foods:
Processed foods can contain high levels of sugar, preservatives, and artificial ingredients that can disrupt the balance of neurotransmitters in the brain, leading to feelings of anxiety and depression.

High-fat and high-sugar foods:
Consuming high levels of sugar and fat can lead to spikes and crashes in blood sugar levels, which can trigger feelings of anxiety and irritability.

Wheat Bran:
Even though experts have been touting wheat bran as a superfood with its high fiber content and complex, nutty flavours, it can significantly increase your anxiety, thanks to its high concentration of phytic acid.

Phytic acid binds to essential mood minerals like zinc and limits their absorption by the body. People who suffer from anxiety need adequate levels of zinc to keep their symptoms at bay.

Soy:
Soy products, while packed with lean protein, is also packed with protease and trypsin inhibitors, which are enzymes that make digesting the protein difficult. Soy products, like tofu, are also high in copper, which is a mineral that has been linked to anxious behaviour.

If you must eat soy, get rid of the tofu and veggie burgers, and try fermented varieties like miso and tempeh, which are much easier to digest.

Coffee:
Coffee is one of the highest concentrated dietary sources of caffeine which can make an anxious brain even worse. Research has shown that people with anxiety disorders are particularly sensitive to feeling the nervous side effects from small amounts of caffeine.

Caffeine can also impede the absorption of vital mood-balancing nutrients like B vitamins and vitamin D.

Whole Wheat Bread:
For many anxious people, gluten is a sticking point, especially with patients who have celiac disease. Most non-organic wheat is treated with an herbicide called glyphosate, which has been shown to cause a nutrient deficiency of mood-stabilizing minerals.

Apple Juice:

Unlike whole apples, apple juice is devoid of the slow-digesting fiber and are often packed with refined fructose.
This results in blood level spikes that can trigger a flood of adrenaline and result in symptoms that look a lot like an anxiety attack. Fructose can actually alter how the brain responds to stress on a genetic level.

Foods that can improve mental health:

Leafy greens:
Leafy greens are high in B vitamins, which are essential for maintaining healthy brain function.

Omega-3 fatty acids:
Omega-3 fatty acids, found in fatty fish and some plant-based oils, can help reduce inflammation and improve mood.

Probiotics:
Probiotics, found in fermented foods such as yogurt and kefir, can help maintain a healthy gut-brain connection.

Whole grains:

Whole grains provide complex carbohydrates that can help regulate blood sugar levels, improving mood and reducing anxiety.

Anxiety isn't a fun condition to have to deal with. However, you can reduce your symptoms and overcome your fear by avoiding these anxiety-inducing foods.

It's important to note that everyone's body is different, and what works for one person may not work for another. However, incorporating a balanced, nutrient-rich diet can have positive impacts on mental health and can help reduce symptoms of anxiety.

Additionally, if you have specific dietary restrictions or concerns, it is best to consult a medical professional or a registered dietitian. They can help you make a personalized nutrition plan that meets your needs and supports your overall health, including your mental health.

The Relationship Between Anxiety and Depression

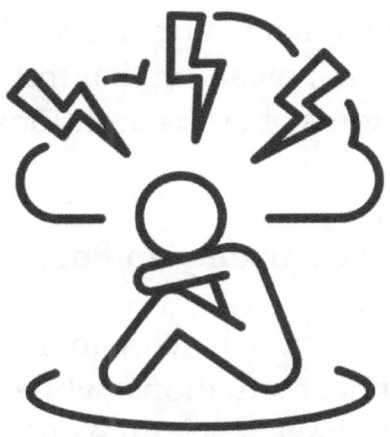

Anxiety and depression are two distinct mental health conditions, but they are often interrelated and can have similar symptoms. This can make it difficult to differentiate between the two.

It is important to understand the similarities and differences between anxiety and depression in order to receive the proper diagnosis and treatment.

Similarities between anxiety and depression:

Symptoms: Both anxiety and depression can cause feelings of worry, fear, sadness, hopelessness, irritability, fatigue, and difficulty sleeping.

Impact on daily life: Both anxiety and depression can have a significant impact on a person's daily life, making it difficult to engage in activities they once enjoyed or to fulfill daily responsibilities.

Comorbidity: Both anxiety and depression are commonly comorbid, meaning that individuals can experience symptoms of both conditions at the same time.

Differences between anxiety and depression:

Focus of worry: Individuals with anxiety tend to worry about future events or situations, while individuals with depression tend to have a negative outlook on life in general.

Physical symptoms: While both anxiety and depression can cause physical symptoms such as fatigue, muscle tension, and headaches, anxiety is more likely to cause physical symptoms such as sweating, palpitations, and shortness of breath.

Onset: Anxiety and depression can have different onset patterns. Anxiety symptoms can develop suddenly in response to a trigger, while depression symptoms may develop gradually over time.

It is important to note that depression is a commonly misrepresented and overused term in relation to a bad mood or negative outlook.

While everyone may experience feelings of sadness or negative thoughts at times, depression is a diagnosable mental health condition that requires professional treatment. Symptoms of depression are persistent, interfere with daily life, and often cannot be improved with positive thinking or self-help strategies alone.

It is important to seek help from a mental health professional if you or a loved one are experiencing symptoms of anxiety or depression, in order to receive a proper diagnosis and effective treatment.

Social Media and Mental Health

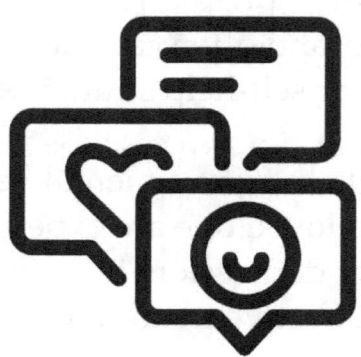

In today's society, social media and marketing have become ubiquitous, shaping our perceptions of ourselves and the world around us.

While these platforms can provide a space for self-expression and creativity, they can also contribute to heightened anxiety and anxiety disorders.

This chapter will explore the impact of social media and marketing on mental health, with a focus on anxiety and anxiety disorders, and provide advice on how to minimise the negative effects and protect ourselves.

Self Esteem Pressure and Societal Pressures:

Social media and marketing often present an unrealistic and idealized view of the world, which can contribute to self-esteem pressure and societal pressures.

The constant exposure to images of perfection, beauty, and success can lead to feelings of inadequacy and low self-esteem. This pressure can be exacerbated by algorithms that tailor content to an individual's interests, leading to a distorted and biased view of reality.
Additionally, social media provides a platform for cyberbullying, further increasing self-esteem pressure and negative body image.

The Impact on Mental Health:

The impact of self-esteem pressure and societal pressures on mental health, particularly anxiety and anxiety disorders, cannot be overstated. Research has shown that the use of social media is directly linked to an increase in anxiety and feelings of hopelessness. The constant exposure to unrealistic and idealised images, combined with the pressure to conform to certain norms, can lead to feelings of stress, depression, and anxiety. In addition, the exposure to negative content, such as cyberbullying and hate speech, can further exacerbate these feelings.

Heightened Anxiety and Anxiety Disorders:
Social media and marketing can contribute to heightened anxiety and anxiety disorders by perpetuating a sense of constant connectedness.

The need to be constantly connected and updated can create a sense of urgency and pressure, leading to feelings of overwhelm and stress. This can trigger symptoms of anxiety, including racing thoughts, panic attacks, and physical symptoms such as sweating, shaking, and headaches. Furthermore, the constant exposure to negative content, such as cyberbullying and hate speech, can increase feelings of anxiety and contribute to the development of anxiety disorders.

Minimising Negative Effects and Protecting Yourself:

To minimise the negative effects of social media and marketing on mental health and protect yourself from heightened anxiety and anxiety disorders, it is important to take a proactive approach. Here are some tips that can help:

1. Limit your exposure to social media and marketing: By limiting the time you spend on social media and marketing; you can reduce the impact it has on your mental health. Try to limit your use to specific times of the day and avoid using it before bed, as it can disrupt your sleep.

2. Unfollow and unfriend negative influences: If you find that following certain people or accounts is causing you stress or negativity, it may be time to unfollow or unfriend them. Surrounding yourself with positive influences can help improve your mental health.

3. Focus on the positive: Instead of dwelling on the negative, try to focus on the positive aspects of social media and marketing. Connect with friends, share your achievements, and engage with others who share your interests.

4. Take a break: If you find that social media and marketing are affecting your mental health, take a break. Go for a walk, read a book, or spend time with family and friends.

5. Practice self-care: It is important to prioritise self-care and prioritise your well-being. This can include engaging in physical activity, practicing mindfulness and meditation, and seeking support from friends and family.

Social media and marketing can have a profound impact on our mental health, particularly our anxiety and self-esteem. By limiting our exposure, practicing self-compassion, seeking out positive and supportive communities, and engaging in self-care, we can minimize the negative effects of social media and marketing and protect our mental health.

Anxiety Disorders In Children

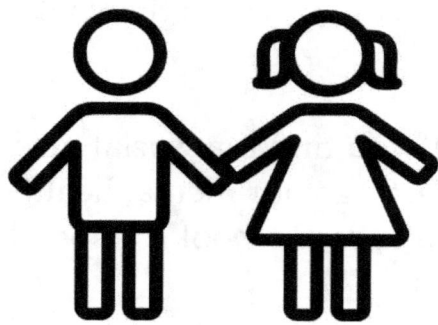

Anxiety disorders are a common mental health concern in children and can have a significant impact on their daily lives.

While some anxiety is a normal part of childhood development, excessive anxiety that interferes with daily activities is a cause for concern. In this chapter, we will explore the contributing factors to anxiety disorders in children, including genetic and environmental factors, as well as the impact of the home environment.

We will also discuss ways for parents and caregivers to protect their child's mental health and provide advice on how to recognize signs of an anxiety disorder.

Genetics:
There is evidence to suggest that anxiety disorders can run in families and may be influenced by genetic factors.

Children with a family history of anxiety or related mental health conditions are more likely to develop anxiety disorders themselves.

Environmental factors:
Environmental factors, such as traumatic experiences or exposure to stress, can also contribute to the development of anxiety disorders in children.

For example, children who have experienced abuse or neglect, or have been exposed to natural disasters or other traumatic events, may be more likely to develop anxiety disorders.

Home environment:
The home environment can also play a significant role in the development of anxiety disorders in children. For example, children who grow up in households with high levels of conflict or stress may be more likely to develop anxiety disorders.

Parental anxiety:
Children who have parents with anxiety disorders are more likely to develop anxiety disorders themselves. This may be due to a combination of genetic and environmental factors, as well as the impact of observing their parents' anxiety.

The Home Environment and Protecting Children's Mental Health:

The home environment can have a significant impact on a child's mental health, and parents and caregivers have an important role to play in creating a supportive and safe environment for their children. Some ways to protect a child's mental health and promote wellbeing include:

1. Providing stability: Providing stability and routine in the home can help children feel safe and secure, reducing their risk of developing anxiety disorders. Establishing predictable schedules and routines can help children feel more in control of their environment and reduce feelings of anxiety.

2. Encouraging open communication: Encouraging open and honest communication can help children feel heard and valued and can also provide an opportunity for parents and caregivers to identify and address any concerns their child may have.

3. Supporting their interests and activities: Supporting children in their interests and activities can help them feel confident and capable and can also provide opportunities for them to develop positive relationships with peers and adults.

4. Modelling healthy coping mechanisms: Modelling healthy coping mechanisms: Modelling healthy coping mechanisms, such as exercise, mindfulness, or seeking support from friends and family, can help children learn effective ways to manage stress and anxiety.

Signs of an anxiety disorder in Children:

Anxiety disorders can be difficult to identify in children, as children may not understand or be able to articulate their feelings. Some signs to look for include:

Physical symptoms: Children with anxiety disorders may experience physical symptoms, such as headaches, stomach aches, or rapid breathing.

Avoidance behaviours: Children may avoid situations or activities that trigger their anxiety, such as going to school or participating in social activities.

Excessive worry: Children may express excessive worry or fear about a variety of situations, such as the future or the safety of loved ones.
Irritability or mood swings: Children may experience.

It is important to seek early intervention from a licensed health care professional if you notice any changes in your Childs mood and / or behaviours that you feel could be a sign that they are struggling with a mental health disorder

Conclusion

I want to take a moment to recognise and applaud you for taking the first step in understanding and managing your anxiety. This journey towards self-discovery and improvement is not an easy one, but I have no doubt that you have the strength and resilience to make it through.

Anxiety can be a challenging and debilitating condition, but with the right knowledge and support, it can be effectively managed. By learning about the different types of anxiety disorders, their causes, and symptoms, you now have a better understanding of what you are facing.

I hope that this book has provided you with a deeper understanding of anxiety, its causes, and how to manage it.

Remember, you are not alone in your struggle with anxiety.

Millions of people around the world face the same challenges as you do.
Taking the steps to educate yourself about anxiety and to seek help is a strong and brave step towards managing your anxiety and taking control of your life. You are capable and strong enough to face these challenges head-on.

By learning about the various triggers, both physical and emotional, and how to manage your thoughts and feelings, you have equipped yourself with the tools necessary to lead a happy and fulfilling life.

And finally, never forget that self-compassion and kindness to yourself is important. Treat yourself with the same kindness and understanding that you would give to someone you love. You deserve to live a life free from anxiety and full of happiness.

As a final reminder, remember the words of Winston Churchill: "Success is not final, failure is not fatal: it is the courage to continue that counts." Just as Churchill did not give up in the face of adversity, neither should you. Keep pushing forward and know that you have the strength within you to overcome anxiety.

www.ingramcontent.com/pod-product-compliance
Lightning Source LLC
Chambersburg PA
CBHW050256220526
45465CB00002B/704